# The Sex Drive Cookbook: Reclaim Your Sex Life by Eating Delicious Foods That Quickly Increase Hormones

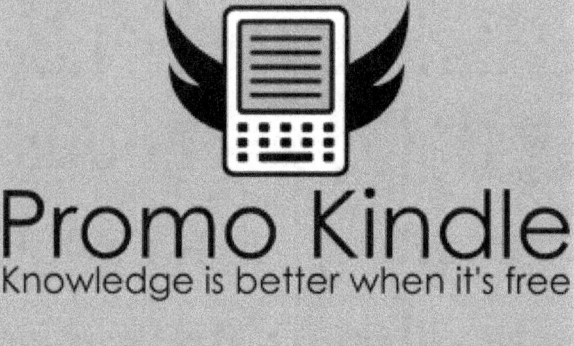

Disclaimer and Terms of Use: Effort has been made to ensure that the information in this book is accurate and complete, however, the author and the publisher do not warrant the accuracy of the information, text and graphics contained within the book due to the rapidly changing nature of science, research, known and unknown facts and Internet. The Author and the publisher do not hold any responsibility for errors, omissions or contrary interpretation of the subject matter herein. This book is presented solely for motivational and informational purposes only.

# Table of Contents

Sexy Betty 34

Sexy Coffee 35

Diva Juice 36

Diablo Diva 37

Pirates Flavor 38

Cherry Liquor 39

Cider 40

Ladies Punch 41

Hot Totty 42

Whether you are going through the "change" or you are just wanting to get a little more action in the bedroom, this is the book for you. Here you will learn about tips to increase your sex drive naturally, what foods to add to the menu, which ones to stay away from, and overall get your groove back.

One thing that both men and women don't take into consideration, is that this is a natural occurrence and believe it or not we will ALL go through it at one time or another. So take a deep breath, don't give up and find your source to get your life back.

# Natural Remedies

You will see a few recipes below that will talk to you about different foods, and recipes that will naturally bring back the libido. But if you don't see anything there that will help fuel your fire, you always can look into figs, bananas and avocados.

## Chocolate ·

Now when did you ever think that chocolate would be something you were encouraged to eat? This is something that will increase the libido, and let's face it, a great treat for everyone!

## The Daily's

Now, if you are someone that takes daily vitamins, you may be missing one of the most important bedroom vitamins. Make sure that you have Gingko Balboa to help treat sexual dysfunction.

It is important to realize that, again, this is something that people suffer from around the globe. With that in mind, take a cue from those in Africa with the yohimbine supplements. This is a form of bark that will help in a more natural form.

Now, it's obvious that sex offers us that feeling of self-confidence, that well, nothing else can offer us. But it is very important that YOU create that feeling of self-worth first. Work on your self-confidence and you WILL be more eager to jump between the sheets.

# Blackberries

# Black Raspberry Shortcake Smoothie

Ingredients:
- 2 C black raspberries
- 1 C crumbled pound cake
- 1 ½ C milk
- 1 ½ C ice

Directions:

Blend in blender and enjoy

# Black Raspberry Mango Smoothie

Ingredients:
- 1 C mango, chopped
- 1 C raspberries
- 1 C coconut milk
- 1 C ice

Directions:

Blend together and enjoy

# Pomegranate Berry Smoothie

Ingredients:
- 1 C black raspberries
- ¾ C beet juice
- ¾ C pomegranate juice
- 1 C ice
- Honey

Directions:

Blend and enjoy

## Spa Sex Fuel

Ingredients:
- 1 lime
- 2 C chopped cucumbers
- ½ C water
- 1 C ice
- 4 T sugar

Directions:

Blend and enjoy

# Black Raspberry Creamsicle

Ingredients:
- ¾ C frozen orange
- ½ C frozen black raspberry
- ½ C cold water
- 1 C vanilla ice cream
- Ice

Directions:

Blend and enjoy

# Honey Raspberry Almond

Ingredients:
- 2 C raspberry
- 1 C almond milk
- Ice
- Honey
- ¼ C chopped almonds

Directions:

Blend and enjoy

# Black Raspberry Vanilla Smoothie

Ingredients:
- 1 pint blackberries
- ½ C raspberries
- 1 C vanilla Greek yogurt
- 1 T honey
- Ice

Directions:

Blend and enjoy

## Pineapple Berry Coconut Smoothie

Ingredients:
- 2 C frozen coconut water
- 2 C chopped pineapple
- 2 C black raspberries
- 1 ½ T lime juice
- 1 T honey

Directions:

Blend and enjoy

# Raspberry Orange

Ingredients:
- ½ C orange juice
- ½ C raspberry juice
- ½ C yogurt
- 1 C ice
- 1 T sugar

Directions:

Blend and enjoy

# Oatmeal Raspberry Cookie Smoothie

Ingredients:

- 1 oats
- 1 C raspberries
- ½ C almond milk
- Ice

Directions:

Blend and enjoy

Broccoli

# Broccoli Coleslaw

Ingredients:
- 1 C olive oil
- 1/3 C white vinegar
- 1/2 C sugar
- 1 pkg. Ramen noodles
- 1 head broccoli, diced
- 2 carrots, sliced
- 1 C chopped onions
- 1 C sunflower seeds

Directions:

I.  Combine everything together in a bowl, and refrigerate overnight
II. Make dressing and pour over broccoli salad when ready to serve

# Tortellini Salad

Ingredients:
- 6 Slices bacon
- 20 oz. package Tortellini
- ½ C mayo
- ½ C sugar
- 2 tsp cider vinegar
- Broccoli, cut up
- 1 C raisins
- 1 C sunflower seeds
- 1 red onion, sliced

Directions:

I. Cook your bacon and crumble, set aside
II. Bring pot of water to a boil and make your tortellini and drain
III. Mix mayo, sugar and vinegar; this will be your dressing
IV. In a separate bowl, mix everything and pour salad dressing over tortellini and toss
V. Serve cold

# Hot Red Salad

Ingredients:
- 2 lbs. bacon
- 1 head broccoli
- ¾ C chopped celery
- 1 ½ C seedless grapes
- ¾ C slivered almonds
- ¼ C white sugar
- 2 T white vinegar
- 1 C mayo
- ¾ C celery
- ¼ C minced onion
- ¼ C red onion

Directions:

I.      Cook bacon, drain and crumble bacon, set aside
II.     Preheat your oven to 300 degrees, and bake your almonds for about 12 minutes
III.    In small bowl, mix everything and toss
IV.     Toss pasta with dressing and broccoli ingredients
V.      Chill in fridge for at least 1-2 hours

## Ranch and Broccoli

Ingredients:
- 1 head broccoli chopped
- Kraft ranch Pasta salad

Directions:

I.      Follow box instructions and add chopped broccoli
II.     Serve

# Broccoli and Cauliflower

Ingredients:
- 1 head broccoli
- 1 head cauliflower
- I can red beans, drained
- 1 can green beans

Directions:

I.      Mix everything together and toss
II.     Refrigerate for 1-2 hours
III.    Serve

Cloves (mix to taste) (Great night cap to get your engine revving!)

# Apple Crunch

Ingredients:
- 1 T Allspice
- 1 T Apple cider
- 1 T Brown sugar
- ½ T Cinnamon
- 1 T Cloves
- 1 C Lemonade
- ½ tsp Nutmeg
- ½ C Orange juice

## Sexy Betty

Ingredients:
- 1 C Ale
- ½ C Brandy
- 1 t Brown sugar
- 1 tsp Cinnamon
- ¼ tsp Cloves
- Lemon wedge
- ¼ C Water

## Sexy Coffee

Ingredients:
- 1 Cinnamon sticks
- 1 T Cloves
- ½ C Coffee
- ½ C Cognac
- 1 Lemon wedge
- 1 Orange/juice
- 2-3 Sugar cubes
- 1 C White curacao

## Diva Juice

Ingredients:
- 1 T Cinnamon
- 1 T Cloves
- 1 C Coffee
- 1 C Dark Rum
- 1 T sugar

## Diablo Diva

Ingredients:
- 1-2 Cinnamon sticks
- 1 T Cloves
- 1 C Coffee
- ¼ C Cognac
- 1 T Cointreau
- 1 T White curacao

## Pirates Flavor

Ingredients:
- 1 T Brown sugar
- 1 tsp Cinnamon
- 1 tsp Cloves
- 1/8 tsp Ginger
- Lemon wedge
- 1 tsp Nutmeg
- 1/2 C Orange juice
- 1/4 C White rum

## Cherry Liquor

Ingredients:
- Cherries
- Cinnamon
- Cloves
- Sugar syrup
- Vodka

# Cider

Ingredients:
- Cider cinnamon sticks
- Cloves
- Sugar

# Ladies Punch

Ingredients:
- 1 tsp Allspice
- 1/4 tsp Brown sugar
- 1 T Butter
- 1/4 T Cinnamon
- 1/8 tsp Cloves
- 1 C Cranberry juice
- Nutmeg
- 1/4 C Pineapple juice
- Salt
- 1/4 C Water

# Hot Totty

Ingredients:
- ½ C Apple juice
- ½ C Apricot Brandy
- 1 Cinnamon sticks
- 1 tsp Cloves

www.ingramcontent.com/pod-product-compliance
Lightning Source LLC
Chambersburg PA
CBHW070844290526
45795CB00002B/977